THE LAST LECTURES

C.G. Jung, 1958

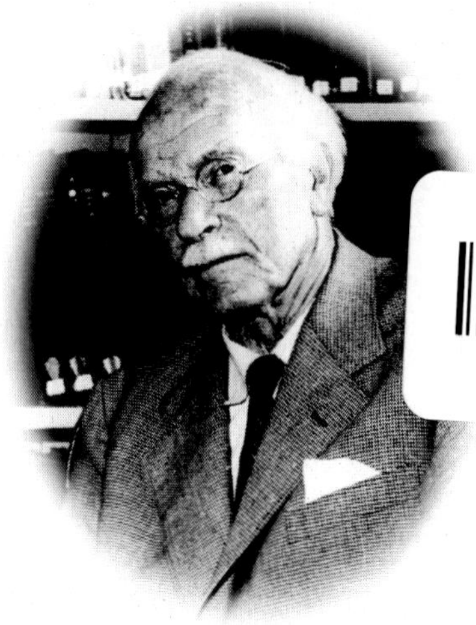

by

C.G. Jung

recollections LLC

CHIRON PUBLICATIONS • ASHEVILLE, NORTH CAROLINA

Translated by Alison Kappes-Bates from *Über Träume und Wandlungen Zürcher Fragestunde* and *Über Gefühle und den Schatten Winterthurer Fragestunden* by C.G. Jung (author), with permission from *The Foundation of the Works of C.G. Jung.*

www.ChironPublications.com

Interior and cover design by Danijela Mijailovic
Printed primarily in the United States of America.

ISBN 978-1-68503-575-4 paperback
ISBN 978-1-68503-576-1 hardcover
ISBN 978-1-68503-577-8 electronic
ISBN 978-1-68503-578-5 limited edition paperback
ISBN 978-1-68503-579-2 limited edition hardcover

Library of Congress Cataloging-in-Publication Data Pending

Acknowledgments

We extend our deepest gratitude to *The Foundation of the Works of C.G. Jung* and Carl C. Jung, whose enduring legacy and vision continue to inspire generations. This publication would not have been possible without their generous permission to share this historic lecture.

Special thanks to Nancy Swift Furlotti, whose work with *Recollections* and her dedication to the integrity of Jung's words have been instrumental in the translation process, and to Alison Kappes-Bates, whose meticulous translation work has helped bring this important material into clear and faithful English.

We are particularly grateful to Murray Stein and Ulrich Hoerni for bringing this extraordinary project to our attention and for recognizing its significance at this moment in time.

With sincere appreciation,

Chiron Publications

Publisher's Note

These original C.G. Jung audio recordings, published for the first time, document legendary informal talks that took place in 1958 at the C.G. Jung Institute Zurich. Addressing an international audience, C.G. Jung responded to selected questions in both German and English on the major themes of his work, but also on many practical aspects of therapeutic treatment. This impressive contemporary document with its relaxed conversational tone provides a very spirited and articulate insight into C.G. Jung's teaching and thinking.

The present text is a transcript of several oral presentations. To preserve its documentary character, it exhibits the characteristics of spoken language. Repetitions, slips of the tongue, pauses, etc. have been moderately eliminated. In some places, the wording could not be definitively determined; here, abbreviations have been made (indicated in the text). Both titles and subtitles of the transcript are editorial additions. Both German and English have their own typography.

The acoustic quality was improved. However, not all the imperfections inherent in a historical document could be corrected. Anyone who listens to the recording should bear this in mind.

Table of Contents

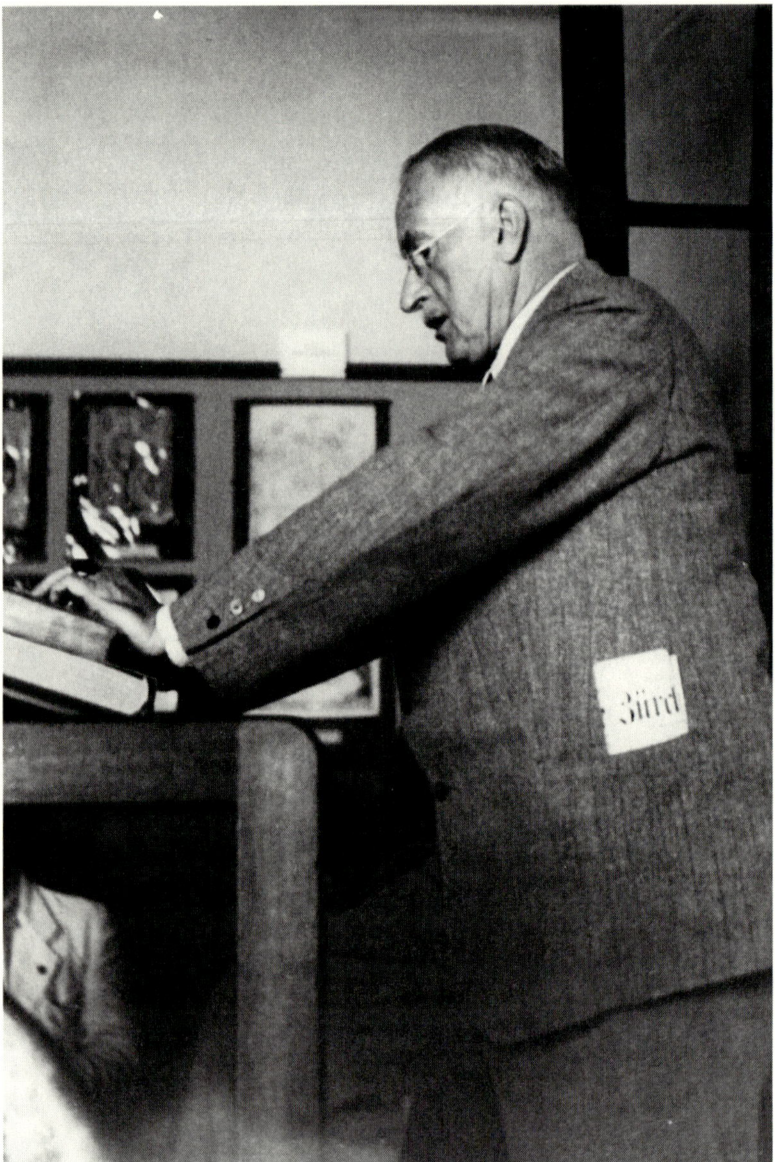

Photo used with permission from *The Foundation of the Works of C.G. Jung.*

Foreword

The circumstances that led to the first publication of these recordings are not fully known. Many who could have provided information remain anonymous, while others may be deceased. From the recollections of a few eyewitnesses as well as from the documents found so far, however, an approximate picture of the creation of the recordings has emerged.

When the C.G. Jung Institute Zurich was founded in 1948, Jung was 73 years old, an age at which one usually likes to retire. Perhaps because of a serious illness that had weakened him in the years before, or perhaps because he wanted to concentrate his energies on important book projects, Jung no longer participated as a lecturer in the Institute that bore his name, and worked only as an advisor and mentor. Among the students—some of whom had come from afar to train in Zurich—there was the natural desire to meet not only Jung's successors but also the man himself. Jung was willing to accommodate their wish. His colloquia with colleagues and friends, often of an interdisciplinary nature, had a long tradition. Two Q&A sessions at the C.G. Jung Institute are documented from 1957, one for members of the Curatorium and one for the students. The first handheld recording and dictation devices also appeared on the market in the 1950's, which made it possible to record conversations in a simple way. The C.G. Jung Institute owned a wire recorder.

The present recordings were made on February 15 and June 14, 1958, and probably on one further date. The participants of the discussions were invited to submit written questions to Dr. Liliane Frey-Rohn, who sifted and forwarded them. A number have been preserved. Some of the questioners summarized their concerns in a few lines, while others sent in several pages of their thoughts. This provided Jung with the opportunity to prepare. He made handwritten notes on individual points. The discussion group met a few days later in the lecture hall of the Psychological Club at Gemeindestrasse 27 in Zurich-Hottingen. Afterwards, tea was served in the rooms of the C.G.

Jung Institute, which were located on the second floor of the same building.

The most well documented event was the Q&A session on June 14, 1958, when, as an eyewitness recalled, the club hall was "very full" (there may have been about 40 people present). She also remembered "how Jung, as always, began dryly, but then became lively and only after an hour and a half, with his face red with excitement, brought the event to a close." Many students at the C.G. Jung Institute were native English speakers. Part of the teaching program was conducted in English. This explains the ease with which both English and German were spoken in meetings. The June 1958 Q&A session was probably the last of its kind. In the fall of 1958, students asked Jung for another meeting with new questions. There is no evidence that this event took place.

At the end of 1959, Jung, by now 84 years old, donated the wire reel recordings to the C.G. Jung Institute "for teaching purposes." Clearly, he found them important for this purpose. The Q&A sessions did not have a single overriding theme. Naturally, most of the questions submitted were of interest to prospective psychotherapists.

Until now, it has been impossible to reconstruct how often the recordings were used after 1959. Jung died in 1961, and in 1979 the C.G. Jung Institute, which by then had grown, moved its headquarters to Küsnacht/ Zurich. In 1988, the attention of the then Director of Studies was once again drawn to the wire recordings that had long since fallen into oblivion.

A functioning playback device no longer existed. Eventually, specialists in English were able to transfer the recordings to tape. Of six reels of wire found, three proved to be rich in content, one was a duplicate, one was fragmentary, and one was unusable. The original wires have since been preserved in the National Sound Archive of the British Library in London.

Ulrich Hoerni

Community of Heirs of C.G. Jung

January 2004

With Gratitude

Not only the audio recordings, but also the preparations undertaken for their publication have a long history. Several people contributed to the success of the project. Thomas Frey, M.D., discovered the wire reels in 1988 and arranged for them to be transferred to tape. Mr. Alistair Bamford supervised the recording at the National Sound Archive. The Curatorium of the C.G. Jung Institute passed various resolutions to approve their publication. From 1992 onward, Dr. Gotthilf Isler was the driving force behind the preparatory work, and it was he who commissioned on behalf of the Foundation for Jungian Psychology Mrs. Margrit Hofmann (dec.) and Mrs. Alison Kappes-Bates to prepare the transcripts. Dr. Gertrud Hess was able to research and reconstruct the circumstances that led to the Q&A sessions. Dr. Wolfram Neubauer permitted the use of archive copies of the ETH-Library Zurich. Mr. Alfred Braun of Bubikon/Zurich oversaw the acoustic preparation of the audio version. We would like to express our gratitude to all the contributors, including those who remain unnamed.

PART 1

ON DREAMS AND TRANSFORMATIONS

ON DREAMS AND TRANSFORMATIONS

The Shadow of Analytical Psychology

[C.G. Jung:]

Ladies and Gentlemen, allow me to address you first in German. I am unable to speak very loudly, so in order to hear me, you must avoid making any background noise. I would like to dive straight in by discussing the questions that have been put to me. The first question—or rather a whole string of questions—was submitted by Mr. Caracciolo. Mr. Caracciolo wants to know what the shadow of Analytical Psychology looks like. As simple as this question sounds, it is almost impossible to answer, for it is so all-encompassing that, if it were to make its way around the world, it would come back to stab Mr. Caracciolo in the back. The shadow that anything casts depends, of course, on what that something is. So, the first question should be: What is Analytical Psychology? And there, I'm out of my depth. I don't know what it is. I only know what it looks like. But what it is, I don't know. That is beyond me. So, it's impossible for me to say anything useful about what this psychology even is. If asked, or if I care to, I can only make statements either about, or on, what the shadow of this statement is. So, first I just think of what its opposite is, or approximately its opposite, for it is immensely difficult to think what the opposite of a complicated thing might be—and of all the things we know, Complex Psychology is among the most complex. Thus, its shadow, too, is extremely complex, so I am unable to outline in a few words what this shadow might be. We would first have to examine each statement precisely and then imagine its opposite, if that were possible. That is also not always possible; one can only think the opposite of relatively simple things. To think the opposite of complicated things is very difficult.

So, after this general introduction, I will now get more specific. The shadow of a complicated thing is, as you have heard, as complicated as the thing itself. For the shadow does not only consist of the light that falls upon something which thereby casts a shadow, but rather it also involves the observer who perceives the thing, who perceives the shadow. And of course, you never know what is being seen because of the projections that are generally, and necessarily, involved. So, if you want to get a general picture of the shadow that is cast by Analytical Psychology—both practically and theoretically—you should just make a list of all the prejudices that are raised in opposition to it when people talk about it. This will give you a very good picture of what Analytical Psychology is when seen from behind. Well, that is most often so, though it is not universally so.

Take any well-defined system whose properties we know by and large, any well-documented mainstream movement—for example the Christian faith which represents the highest ideal—and ask about its shadow. Indeed, you might say that behind Christianity is hell's scornful mockery. And if you want to get more theoretical—if one could—than what people say or what happens, and consider what constitutes its shadow, you would not be able to fathom what its opposite would be from the documented content of the Christian religion; it's impossible; it's too complex. But you can rest assured that such an isolated position which [such] a complex represents could not possibly exist without casting a shadow, for otherwise it would not exist at all. Everything that exists casts a shadow, and thus, for example, the actual shadow of Christianity that exists is a tremendous shadow—a terrible and tragic shadow; I would say, it is a jeering from hell.

And of course, the same holds true for psychology. Quite apart from the faults inherent in everything, the positive outcomes of any man-made thing are inherently brought about by the opposites. You cannot adopt a standpoint without some negative resulting from it; it is simply a part of it, for otherwise it is not real. Naturally, one can scrutinize this psychology for its faults. My entire life's endeavor has been to look for where the weak points are, for where the contradictions lie, and [I] have tried to eradicate them, to tweak things until they more or less work. Many things are difficult to formulate; it is, after all, an empirical matter, and one can get the wording of things wrong. Naturally, I had to make changes to some of my terms and definitions. I have had to modify many of my views over the course of my life, which is inevitable. What has emerged is not perfect, of course, but I wouldn't know where to make any fundamental changes. What I do know is that, empirically speaking, when the entire edifice makes its appearance out in the world, a tremendous shadow emerges, which is as real as the thing itself. And insofar as you are identified with this psychology, you are, of course, trapped within this shadow. If you don't want to be caught in it, you must find out where you can improve on it, and if you do improve on it, you'll then be caught by that special shadow because of what you did. [Laughter] Nothing a human being comes up with is completely good, for then it wouldn't be real—*nolens, volens*, a shadow effect arises. But there is little point in going into detail, for I don't know where the main errors lie; they will appear over time, but I don't know them yet. If I knew them, I would have worked on them. I have never imagined that I had managed to shoot down the whole bird. There are still plenty of questions to work on, for instance, the whole historical question, the comparative question, the connection with biology, and so on. Indeed, it's riddled with holes.

But if no one works on it seriously, there is no one there to fill these holes. And if someone were to fill these holes, then they would have to deal with reality, for they would have fallen into the shadow that was cast when they did something good and new. This is very dangerous; steer clear of this if you can! Being a pioneer is no fun. For you may not forget that if you manage to have a single new and good thought (or a bad one, but nevertheless a new one), then you are the only person who has had that thought, and you will pay for it. For then you are alone, and you cannot help but identify with this new thought. For this is your truth which you have happened upon and to which you commit yourself with all of who you are, if you are worth your salt in the first place; and then you are completely isolated, for you will fall into the shadow of this thing.

Now, if you are in a position—as indeed you are—to familiarize yourself with this psychology, you will inevitably be presented with results; you will hear concepts and viewpoints which you will take in as words spoken by the teacher. Initially, you will have trouble understanding these words, to grasp what could be meant by them. At first, you will understand these words roughly as follows: You are told that this is how it is, so you must talk about it as if it were so, or as if you were convinced that it was like this, or as if you knew it were thus. But you know only words; you have no idea what the reality is; you know only the words on such and such a page.

I once saw an intelligent colleague who pestered me

with all kinds of questions, and I asked him what he had read of mine. This was many years ago, and he had read, for example, *The Transformations and Symbols* book—*Symbols of Transformation* and [my book on] typology. And then we analyzed a dream, and I referred to the latter—to the theory of functions, etc.—and he had understood nothing at all, not a word. So, I said, "Yes, but you told me you'd read my book on typology." And he said, "I have indeed read it, but what you're telling me has nothing at all to do with that." Then I said, "Well, please, have a look: there, there and there. It's perfectly clear that it's about thinking, about feeling, about intuition, etc." He hadn't seen that at all. I then questioned him as to how he had read my typology book, and finally he said, "Well, I actually thought that it was all just words!" So, you see, he had only read the words and had not made the slightest effort to imagine what it might mean if someone thinks like that, or if someone sees things in that way. He had merely committed words to memory.

So, at first, all you can do is memorize words and be preoccupied with concepts. And the less you have understood about a matter, the more you will be preoccupied with concepts, for that is all you have.

You have nothing other than concepts and words to defend yourself with, without at all having grasped the thing itself. If you have mentally grasped anything at all, it has remained stuck in the linguistic region, just there… but it has not penetrated your whole being. In psychology, you have only understood a thing when you have lived it, or when it has entered the realm of doing and experiencing, but not before.

So, initially you simply learn how to hold a hammer or a pair of pliers, but you have not yet made a hammer or a pair of pliers. And that's what it's all about, namely that a word penetrates the depth of one's being, where it truly becomes who we are, and we live within it. When that happens, when you go beyond just words, when you move down from the Kundalini Châkra Vishuddha, to at least the region of Anâhata, to the heart and lung region, once you have come that far, you know what the heart has to say about it and what the mind has to say about it. But you are still only in the intellect, which still means nothing at all.

But if you can press on into greater depths, which is inevitable if you hear the word, if you really hear it, i.e., if you allow it to penetrate you, then you will fall within the ambit of the shadow that is attached to this thing. Then you yourself become affected by the shadow, and this is a very difficult problem, for then it is as if you were the originator of this thing, i.e., you are then in my position and will discover that you are isolated. You are isolated from humanity; you are not only isolated from the herds of blockheads, but also from the intelligent people who have a different viewpoint or, particularly where psychology is concerned, have preconceived ideas.

And no one can avoid this. Like anyone who has a new idea, you are then in a very disagreeable situation. This is why I believe you must make anyone who has a new idea aware of the psychological consequences; otherwise, people are terribly surprised when they suddenly realize that they are no longer at home anywhere—except in Zurich. And usually, one has the unfortunate habit of clinging to like-minded people. This is necessary, of course, but it creates a spiritual inbreeding, and it is done to protect oneself from this isolation. The only chance of survival for many people is if they can assure themselves of some support, as it were, at the very least the spiritual support of like-minded people. And this is then a womb, a spiritual womb, in which one quietly stays put, to prevent having to expose oneself to the dangers of life. For, as soon as they encounter the world at large, they are immediately at risk. Mr. Caracciolo has very correctly called this experience—this identification with words—a pseudo-victory, which it is.

So, if you ever engage with psychology, or allow yourself to be moved by it in a way that has fateful consequences, only then do you really begin to feel the effect of it; until then you are for the most part, forgive me, made stupid by it. You will only be intelligent when you have put yourself on the line for it in the world, and that only because you had to. This is the great disadvantage of a new and unpopular idea, and of course you cannot afford to have any illusions about this by thinking, for example, that because it is psychology, you will be welcomed; by individuals, perhaps, but not in the main, because the world is very different from the way we try to imagine it. If this were not so, the world would be in a different state to what it currently is.

So now I would like to ask if anyone has any comments on this, or a question? Well, if that is not the case, then—Yes, please?

[Question:] In relation to this new idea, I wanted to ask how you understand "idea" here. I have. . . to my way of thinking, I have often thought, I don't generate ideas, but rather, speaking now from my own experience, I enter-into-a-relationship with an eternal idea, which then determines me. And I simply wanted to ask you how you understand this 'idea.' I also believe that by entering-into-a- relationship with an idea, the human being is somehow opened to a greater experience ...

[C.G. Jung:] Yes, yes….

[Question:] ... and not closed, isolated, but rather more the opposite.

[C.G. Jung:] I just now used the term idea, but I could as well have said that I became acquainted with a new fact; it's exactly the same, in practical terms. So, for example, if I live in a world where there are no bacteria, then it is a new experience for me, a very impressive experience, that drinking water can be infected with typhoid. This completely changes how I see the world. Now that is simply a fact, but it is simultaneously also an idea. You say to yourself, "Well, this water could be infected." You don't drink it or give it to other people to drink. That's a new idea, because previously I thought it was completely harmless. Or, for example, take the relationship of children to a submissive mother or a tyrannical father: both have always existed, but the new idea or new fact is that one knows, for example, that a mother's submission can be an extremely dangerous thing—a thought one had not had previously; or that the tyranny, the so-called tyranny, of the father is, under certain circumstances, a very desirable thing, for the children lack a paternal influence. America! Children need to be educated; they need to be shaped, and of course they want to kick against that, which is their prerogative. But fathers must be able to enforce their will, because that is what children expect; otherwise, everything gets out of hand. The increase in juvenile delinquency in America is simply appalling. Psychology in America is gradually *cocking its ears* because it is becoming worrisome.

[A female voice:] Would you mind answering an English question?

[C.G. Jung:] Well, if you want to speak English, don't be afraid [laughter]—if you have understood what I said before. Otherwise, I am unable to tell the whole story once more in English. I can only tell you that Mr. Caracciolo asked about the shadow cast by analytical psychology in general. My view is that it casts a tremendous shadow which you can see if you open your eyes. You can read it everywhere, but one could not construct a real, a valid shadow by the data, by the documentary data, given by analytical psychology because I simply don't know where the great holes are. I always try to fill them, and as far as I have seen them, I have filled them as well as possible. Of course, it is not perfect; I have done it as well as I could. It is up to the critics to do better. No question? All right, then we go on.

The Fourth Dimension - Symmetry and Asymmetry

[C.G. Jung:] Here is a question, Mr. Kirsch, which I cannot fully answer; it is too specific. You ask about the fourth dimension in my little book on the modern myth. The relation of the asymmetry of the image[1] to the asymmetry problem of modern nuclear physics is one of those analogies, of which there are quite a

[1] Jung is referring here to the picture "The Fourth Dimension" by Peter Birkhäuser in *CW 10*, §736-747, fig.3.

few, between the psychology of the unconscious and nuclear physics. This analogy must arise because both sciences—of course, in a completely different way—approach the unknown, and the unknown is the same everywhere, namely it is unknown. Whether you say "unconscious" and mean something psychic, or whether you say "unknown" and mean something physical, the fact that you mean something does not improve the thing; it is simply unknown.

When I say there is something unknown going on in this country, it can be something physical or something psychological; we do not know what it is. Consequently, when we start speculating about this unknown in an absolute way, it is not at all clear whether this is psychic or physical; we apply the same categories. So that's why, for example, in the latest speculations in nuclear physics there is matter and anti-matter, and as the basis of the world there is a universon—a terrible word. Now that is just pure mythology. So, this is what the concept of asymmetry is saying, or is on the way to saying, isn't it? The concept of asymmetry is the concept of parity: the right side is the same as the left side, only it's on the right.

Well, symmetry—you could almost say the axiom of symmetry—in physics is also not a statistical truth, but it was thought that symmetry, too, was, so to speak, almost axiomatic. And now, because of the so-called Chinese Puzzle—do you know what that is? You don't? These are the two Chinese who discovered the left-handedness of the mesons; this is the so-called Chinese Puzzle. They found out that most of the mesons—they had already counted around 50,000 observations at the time—they found out that the mesons are mainly left-handed. And Pauli, Professor Pauli, told me that the conclusion that could be drawn from this is that the Good Lord must be slightly left-handed. [Laughter] Well, we also have this question of symmetry in psychology, namely that shadows and consciousness are a parity: they are complementary, or compensatory. But the concept of compensation only comes into it because there is no real parity, but rather an asymmetry. It is not completely symmetrical, for if it were, things would have come to a complete standstill long ago. For symmetry always works towards being identical, with the only difference being that one is on the right, the other on the left, but both are present. In which case, nothing would ever happen. It must be asymmetrical; it must…it can never quite fit, which is why things keep rolling on; [otherwise] things wouldn't keep rolling.

And this is the same in psychology. If I had been able to talk about it, I would have said, "Yes, of course we must postulate an asymmetry, for otherwise we would already be in a state of suspension, because of symmetry." Symmetry cannot sustain life, so if the psyche is presently still alive, there must then be an asymmetry. Thus, psychological considerations are completely in line with the physical ones, i.e., being is not symmetrical; being is not static; being is an unstable equilibrium—because of asymmetry. I can't say much more about it, about the physical side anyway, for I am not competent, and I can't say much about the psychological side either, for there, things are too subtle. I know too little about it. I've only hinted at it. Do you have any further questions about this?

The Developmental Capacity of the Human Being

[C.G. Jung:] Now we come to the next question, Dr. Hess. This is the question: * -

*[Dr. Gertrud Hess:] "Can one conclude from your statement [that mankind is in its youth] that humankind

is essentially still capable of development? On what basis can we conclude that we are not approaching the end of time, but are merely in a process of transformation?"

I once made a remark that humankind is still very young and… which means that it is still capable of development. Of course, I mean this from the psychological standpoint where it is our experience that the individual is capable of development, and if some individuals are capable of development, we can perhaps jump to the conclusion that all of them, or at least, let's say, 51%, have this same capacity for development. I do not mean, of course, a physical capacity for development, but rather a psychological one.

If I were to unjustifiably conclude that because a certain number of individuals prove to be psychologically capable of development—implying that this capacity for development would also be inherited, in the sense of inherited characteristics—this would, of course, be nonsense. We have no confirmation that the acquirements or developments that parents undergo are passed on to their children; this goes without saying. It always starts anew.

This assertion of mine that humankind is still in its youth is based, on the one hand, on the biological fact that mankind appeared relatively late on the tree of development, that is, as the *genus homo sapiens*, and, on the other hand, that individuals still prove themselves to be capable of development: they can, for example, develop a kind of adaptation that they or their environment did not previously have. In the psychic realm, the capacity to develop is present. And by humankind I did not really mean humankind from the biological standpoint; I could have as easily said "the public," which in many respects is still exceedingly infantile. I certainly do not need to give you examples; you have only to read the newspapers and study what is going on in politics. It is so unimaginably infantile, it is horrifying, and there is still a lot that could be developed into much better forms.

Now Dr. Hess asks whether we can conclude from this that we are not approaching the end of time but are merely in a process of transformation. Well, I am not able to draw such a conclusion, for I simply do not know if we are approaching the end of time or if we are in a process of transformation. Many things are changing, but whether this will lead to the end or to a new beginning, nobody knows. I spoke of the end of time, but only in the sense of the Platonic year, namely that in the Platonic year typical transformations occur which correspond to the sections of the precession of the vernal equinox, which we know especially from Egyptian history or from the psychology of Christianity. Any questions?

[G. Hess:] So you would say that one doesn't know whether humankind will ever mature? One doesn't know?

[C.G. Jung:] Well, one doesn't know; that's impossible.

[G. Hess:] So whether humanity will ever become peaceful, that is, a mature humanity that is at peace . . .

[C.G. Jung:] Dear me, that's a remote ideal; that's like a good intention that paves the road to hell. [Laughter] Those speculations are too far-reaching for me.

One more question, perhaps? If not, then I'll go to the next one.

PART 2

ABOUT THE ANIMUS

ABOUT THE ANIMUS

[C.G. Jung:] Ms. Heumann asks: Is the animus of a woman whose superior function is thinking in possession of her feelings, and producing inferior value judgements, or is her superior thinking due to her developed animus, while the Eros principle remains unconscious and in the hands of the shadow?

When the animus of a woman whose superior function is thinking is in a normal condition, then there is no reason whatever why she shouldn't or couldn't be in possession of her feelings. When her thinking functions properly, it will not interfere with her feeling values and so it will not stop her feeling development; on the contrary, it will lead to it. Because when you follow your intellectual development, you will soon come to a place where fate will show you that you can't get by with intellect alone, that you need feeling. You cannot go on within that development and not get into a collision with your feeling values. Your intellectual development would be badly at fault if you neglect those values. Not that this hasn't happened: that is just our trouble: we develop our intellect with no regard to feeling values and then you simply become stupid, dumb, as intellectual people who neglect feeling values are. Nothing is more stultifying than the absence of feeling values.

Now it is true that when a woman has a superior thinking function, she has probably developed her thinking through the critique of her own animus. That would be necessary, for no thinking can be developed under the influence of an animus, because the animus is the opposite of thinking. For example, I criticize a woman and then she says, "Oh, I thought . . ."—which means she did *not* think. [Laughter] You see? Because when she says, "I thought," she did not think; she was being thought by her animus; she had an animus opinion. For example, I say to her, "Now look here, I dislike when you do this or that." Then she does it and then I say, "Now why did you do that?" "Oh, I thought you liked it." [Laughter]

You see? That is what the animus does, even down to the smallest detail. For example, you say, "Oh, are you going to the shop? Could you bring me a little box of cigars of that and that kind, but only a little one?" Then she brings me a big one, because I said a little one. [Laughter] And then she says, "Oh! I thought…." So, you see, for her to have a superior intellect, she must have gone through a process of cleansing [her] intellect, because the animus is absolutely prohibitive. The animus is not the mind: it is the very opposite of real intellect. But, you see, if on the other hand her superior thinking is a superior animus, then her real intellect is inferior. Her intellect, or what appears to be her intellect, is nothing but her animus. Then she possesses no intellect. Behind the screen, the screen of her animus, she can be as stupid as you please, and this she is. I shall never forget: I was once at a diplomatic dinner and the lady I was afflicted with [laughter] was the sister of a very famous man. She was apparently *the* big thing, the big mind, and she moved in a very intellectual circle. From the moment we sat down, for one and a half hours, she absolutely swamped me with philosophy and God knows what. I had no chance to get in a single word. Then suddenly she stopped, feeling that now I must be floored, and said, "But I always talk. What are *your* views?" with reference to this or that—highly abstruse philosophical subjects. I said, "You know, I would be very interested to know what you think about these things." "But I have just swamped you with my ideas!" To which I said, "No madam, you haven't. You told me only what I could read in the *Encyclopedia Britannica.* [Laughter] I am not interested in all that stuff. I would like to know what you think." "What *I* think? Oh well, then I should have to think about it first." [Laughter]

Well, the result was that the next day she called me up and wanted to see me privately for a consultation. [Laughter] She had discovered that she had never thought the slightest thing in the world. That is a superior animus. But everybody swears she is the most intelligent, extraordinary, educated person. She only talks drivel, intellectual drivel; she knows nothing; she has acquired nothing. It's all talk. That should be a superior intellect!

Now such an animus, such a sort of quasi-intellect, is most prohibitive where the development of feeling is concerned because it kills the feeling completely, not only the feeling of her public, but also her own feeling. Her own feeling remains very primitive and helpless, lame, ridiculous, childish, egotistical; her feeling is simply impossible. And she is also unable to establish a feeling rapport because her feeling has been killed from the start. You see, when a woman begins to talk such drivel, a man with any trace of intelligence simply drifts off; he falls asleep. [Laughter] As a matter of fact, I had the greatest trouble not to fall asleep, and the only thing that kept me alive was eating and drinking. [Laughter] Any other question?

[Question:] Dr. Jung, would you equate the intellect with her thinking conscious ...

[C.G. Jung:] Yes, yes, with her thinking conscious.

[Question:] ... or with the speculative and practical side of the intellect which goes into ego cognition?

[C.G. Jung:] No, no, you can find the definition of intellect in my *Psychological Types*—it is the function of thinking, whatever that is. But only philosophers don't know what thinking is; psychologists do! [Laughter] Any other question?

[Question:] Could one say that superior...

[C.G. Jung:] A bit louder, please.

[Question:] ...that superior thinking is not due to a superior animus but to a redeemed one? Would that be right?

[C.G. Jung:] What? The superior intellect?

[Question:] Yes.

[C.G. Jung:] The real one?

[Question:] ... is due to a redeemed animus?

[C.G. Jung:] Not due to a redeemed animus, but that the redemption of the animus is due to better thinking. That woman I spoke of only gets rid of her animus when she begins to think. When she condescends enough to come down to the fact that she has never thought and she does not know what thinking is; then she begins, and *that* is the redemption of the animus. The animus is caught in its own primitivity. You see, that is the spirit that fell into matter and must be liberated. That can only be done by real thinking, by the thinking of the individual, not by that demon that consists chiefly of words. This is, of course, the danger for any woman with a good intellect: that she eats the wrong food, that she eats the straw and not the oats, the husks and not the contents.

And of course, there are men who cater to it, men whose whole intellect consists of words. They use words as a sort of magical means to twist the mind of women. You see that in practical cases of *fils à papa* where the father produces the wrong kind of spirit, and she eats all that and is poisoned for a lifetime.

Now of course, what I have said here about these misadventures in a woman's development is equally valid for men. There you see the same twisting of the feeling life of a man through the viciousness of the sloth or the lies of the mother.

Now there is Mr. Rhally's question. I'd better read it: "When we speak of repression, does this imply that the repressed matter once arose to a conscious level from its origin, in which case the difference between suppression and repression would be a matter of the *present* degree of consciousness, or is it possible for repression to function without the repressed matter ever having come up to consciousness?"

Now this is quite an apt problem which, when I was quite a young man and still a good friend of Professor Freud, I took up with him. The term repression confers the idea that a content, which must be a conscious content—otherwise you couldn't speak of it—is repressed by an action, say a moral action or something like that, that is equally conscious. But then I made my association experiments, and I found complexes that had never been conscious, couldn't have been conscious, and they were repressed. So, the conundrum arose: the patient had never been conscious of this fact, yet it showed itself in a repressed state. He never repressed it; he never knew it. Something, then, has developed within him from his unconscious and he didn't know that such a development had taken place. It is all quite naturally in an unconscious state; it is subliminal; it hasn't reached the surface yet; it was never on the surface to be repressed.

I put that question to Freud, and he said, "Yes, you are quite right. There are such things." But he never made use of it. Later on, I came back to it, and he didn't like it because that was a case that made the theory of repression inapplicable. It is awkward, isn't it, when one has such a nice theory of repression that applies in most cases and suddenly you have a case where it doesn't apply. For an explorer, that is a most lamentable fact: he has built up a nice conception of something and he has all the legitimations for it and suddenly discovers that it doesn't apply in every case where it should. Of course, one dislikes it, but I always felt a sort of defeat when it happened to me. That perhaps there is a world of experiences that doesn't apply to the concept which was meant to catch them.

I can well remember the time when I was revising the types. I first thought only of thinking and feeling types. Then—by chance, I should say—I discovered that sensation must play a role. I thought, "Well of course, but sensation is not thinking, and it is not feeling, so we have three functions." Now I have to say, we have two functions: we have extraverts and introverts. Feeling is extravert and thinking is introvert. That's absolutely pat, you know. And then along comes that little hell of sensation [laughter] and overthrows my whole applecart. Naturally I hate it; I would have hated it more if a young person had told me, "But aren't you overlooking sensation?" Of course I would have hated it. That's hellishly awkward because every man who is doing research work is vain regarding his work. He is terribly vain that he has such a nice mistress, or that he has a nice hat, or that he has written a nice book; and so he cannot go back on it. Finally, it is shown that it is not so marvelous after all. Well, that's hateful.

So naturally I was particularly careful to examine whether it is really legitimate for sensation to be a function. Today, I would say it is perfectly ridiculous to make any bones about it. Of course it is a function.

Then, mind you, I didn't know about intuition. That was the last because it is, of course, also the most difficult. Because it really has no proper estimation: it is not rational. It is rational to think, that is, to want to know what a thing is. It is also quite rational to know or to learn what a thing is worth to you. It is also, after all, quite rational to state that a thing exists, which is sensation. And then what? You see, there is nothing beyond that, and so I say we have three functions. And lo and behold, I had a patient, an intelligent lady who was quite clever in certain ways, but highly neurotic. One day she said to me, "Why don't you speak of intuition?" I said, "What do you mean by intuition? That is not a function." It was not in my three functions, you see. What is intuition after all? It's a hunch. That's nothing. How can you define an intuition? Intuition pops into your mind. You are suddenly reminded of something; you foresee a certain thing which you couldn't possibly foresee. It's most illegitimate, you see, most illegitimate. How can you know something ahead? Nobody knows anything ahead. It is just guesswork. An English professor who wrote a very scientific criticism of Rhine's ESP said, "All those recognitions and all that ESP function—that's nothing but guessing!" [Laughter] He thought it was a big deal, saying it was nothing but guessing. So, I said, "Oh, that's nothing but a lucky guess, or something. It is not a function." But you see, what that lady said had given me quite a jolt. And then I began to pay attention. I began to study what intuition is, and then I discovered how it works, and then I knew, "Aha!" She was an intuitive, of course. I studied her very carefully, and when I saw a certain expression appearing on her face, I knew: now she is intuiting. [Laughter] That expression was a sort of bland expression that one couldn't make out. She was simply staring at and through, and then I knew: now she is going to say something, and so it was.

If you want to know what I mean by that peculiar look, look at the picture of Goethe by Stieler. There he's got the intuitive eye. You see, I observed that face in all its phases. At the same time, I had a patient who was a sensation type, a very accurate and objective observer of things just as they are. Now the two became acquainted and he occasionally invited her for a little ride in a boat on the lake. There they noticed these divers, these birds on the lake, and they began a game, namely, to guess where the diver would come up again and who would be the first to see it. He lost every bet: she was always ahead of him. The one who was not aware of reality to an uncanny degree always saw the bird coming up first. He lost every bet because he did it in the legitimate way of observing: you just watch out; you look for where the bird might come up. She did nothing of the sort: she didn't observe at all; she had it in her bones. Now explain that.

But I saw it is a function. It does exist but it is something like ESP, and that is not allowed in decent society. [Laughter] So I am up against it.

That was my first defeat. There the great shadow began because I admitted the existence of intuition. Which is really an obscenity because it cannot be. It shouldn't be. Somebody who does not observe observes better than a trained observer. Which is a fact.

Now I don't know how I got to this. How did I get to this argument about the four [laughter] functions?

[Question:] I would like to go back to that...

[C.G. Jung:] Yes.

[Question:] ... because it was a question of repression ...

[C.G. Jung:] Yes, yes, yes.

[Question:] ... suppression or repression, and how one would ...

[C.G. Jung:] No, repression, repression.

[Question:] ... and how one would explain these contents which have never been conscious and yet were obviously repressed.

[C.G. Jung:] Well, when a thing was never conscious then it cannot be a question of conscious suppression. You see, repression as Freud seems to understand it would really be a suppression because there is a will to suppress. But you know, he is not quite clear about it. As far as I remember our talks about it, I always had the impression… as if he meant something he is not exactly doing, that it sort of happened to him. And that is of course the superego about which there was no question in those days—it didn't exist then.

So you see, his concept of repression always had a little bit of something involuntary. It just happened, somehow. One found out that [it was] because the father had said so and so, or because you read in the bible that you don't do it, or it is wrong. So, he never took full responsibility for that term or the fact of repression. For example, take the censor in the dream, which is the same, you know. The censor happens in the dream. It functions in the dream where one is not properly conscious, and one cannot say that you are the censor. But the censor is, and [it] prevents one from dreaming something obscene or incompatible. I had that discussion, too, with Dr. Freud personally. I said, "I admit if you dream of a revolver, of a rifle, of a walking stick, of a church spire that this can be a phallic symbol. But when you dream of a real penis, what then?" "Ah, then the censor hasn't functioned." [Laughter] So, the censor is an autonomous figure, a very mystical something. And later, it became obvious that it was the superego. But in those days [when] I was with Freud, that concept didn't exist. So, his idea of repression remained a bit in the dark. But when we speak of his theory, I would rather use the word suppression: "I know this is wrong, therefore it must go." Or as Nietzsche says, "This is what I have done; I cannot have done it; I cannot do—I could not have done such a thing!"[1] Finally, memory fades out, which means it is no more. Now you see, that is how repression works. But this is when you pull it out into the light. Then you must say, "Well, for such and such reasons, I am quite conscious of not having thought about the decalogue[2]. I had my education, and for those reasons I exclude this thing. I let it drop off the table, or I stamp my foot upon it." It would then be unconscious up there.

In contrast to these repressions, there are things that are definitely not repressed because they are utterly unconscious. They begin to germinate in the unconscious; they reach a certain level in the unconscious and suddenly they pop up and there it is. They have never been repressed because one never knew them. If you assume that the repression works unconsciously, then you would be confronted with the fact that a thing you don't know is suppressed by a thing of which you know nothing. Now how is that possible? Because when everything is in

---

[1] In one English translation, the citation Jung is quoting reads: **"I did that," says my memory. "I could not have done that," says my pride, and remains inexorable. Eventually – memory yields.** (F. Nietzsche, *Beyond Good and Evil*, Aphorism 68.)
[2] The Ten Commandments.

the unconscious, you are just not conscious of it, and so you cannot say something is happening there, because you don't know. So, the hypothesis that repression works by itself, as it were, that the contents are unknown, the repression, the fact is unknown—is an assumption on your part that there is such a thing. In fact, you know nothing. You know neither the repressor nor the repressed, so we must dismiss that possibility.

[C.G. Jung:] There is, for example, a question from Dr. Spiegelman about the symbol and its distinction from the sign. Now that is a theme you know and probably are well-informed about, and it can be found practically everywhere. That's an elementary thing which doesn't need a special answer.

On the other hand, there is the question whether a main symbol that shapes your life is necessarily unconscious. That is not the case, not at all: it is not necessarily unconscious. It can be highly conscious. Think, for example, of the Christian symbol or any other. The bringing up to consciousness of an unconscious symbol doesn't settle that symbol or empty it of its contents. On the contrary, it can stay on, of course, as long as it does not age. That means, for as long as it *expresses the underlying constellation*. When *that* changes over the course of time, perhaps over a long [period of] time, then it ages, and then it does not express any more, neither totally nor partially. Now the idea of synchronicity has nothing to do with projection, with psychological projection; those two concepts are incommensurable.

The Individuation Process of So-called "Simple" People

Now we come to another question, namely—excuse my smoking, but after life, it shall cease. Now this is a German question from Monsieur Caracciolo:

"How does the individuation process unfold in people who know nothing about psychology, in so-called normal, or better, 'simple' people? I assume that as a spontaneous and natural process, the individuation process also takes place in these people. Is it, perhaps, more likely that this process takes place in such people through certain collective experiences, attitudes, and symbols?"

I have often been asked this question in the belief that the individuation process is, as it were, a therapeutic measure that the physician uses to relieve a patient of their neurosis. Of course, this is not the case at all. The individuation process is something every being can do. If you plant an acorn in the ground, an oak tree will grow, and if a tiger has a cub, it will become a tiger and not a head of lettuce. The individuation process is a natural process that takes place everywhere, and if you want to study it in its natural simplicity, just go to the primitives, and there you will see the individuation process in all its splendor.

I have brought a book along for you, a new book[3] about the *Naskapi Indians* in Labrador. They believe that everyone has the Great Man within them. This idea is characteristic of Chinese philosophy. There, it is the *Chên-yên*, the complete man, the whole man, the perfect man, the ultimate man, i.e., what the alchemists called the *homo quadratus*, the square man, the real man. And, incidentally, they write: "The great man reveals itself in dreams; every individual has one and in consequence has dreams." Those who respond to their dreams by paying them

[3] Frank G. Speck: *Naskapi: The Savage Hunters of the Labrador Peninsula.*

serious attention, by thinking about them and by trying to interpret their meaning in secret and testing out their truth, can cultivate deeper communication with the Great Man. He then sees qualitatively better. The next obligation is for the individual to follow the instructions given in dreams and to memorialize them in representations of art, like, for example, a mandala divided into four parts, as we know it from our analytical work where we have encountered it hundreds of times. Well, there you have the individuation process in a nutshell.

Interestingly, the author says that this Great Man is obviously the ego. Well, he's practically a modern scientist, isn't he, when he alleges such nonsense, for he can't yet distinguish between what is me and what is it. These primitives say quite clearly that the Great Man—the square man, *homo quadratus*—is in everybody, and it is from him that dreams come. They do not say that dreams come from the ego, but from *him*. And they say the «Great Man» because everyone feels themselves to be small. The primitives I talked to were so humble they even said that no one has big dreams, that dreams have no meaning at all, and that they have no dreams. I said, "Why do you say that? You have dreams, don't you?" Then they said, "It's not important. The medicine man or the chief, the headman, *he* has dreams."

So, these are the big dreams of the tribe; these are the mana personalities. The chief is mana, and the medicine man is mana, and *they* have the big dreams. But the ordinary person, the ordinary human being, has no dreams, no dreams at all; there's no mention of them at all. Well, that shows how highly they value dreams and what it means when someone has mana. *Nun, diese Leute da, das sind Indianer, die sind ein bisschen weiter wie meine Neger, die waren viel zu primitiv.*[4] But this is a higher state, a universal concept of everybody having the Great Man within, and clearly, this is the Chên-yên of Chinese philosophy, which is an ancient Mongolian connection from the migration of peoples from the Indus Valley. There you can see that it is the Great Man who bestows dreams, which is why you must listen to your dreams. And the dreams are *a deo*

[4] This sentence literally translates into "These people are Indians, who are a little bit more advanced than my negroes, who were much too primitive." The modern reader may be taken aback by the use of such words, which were common in the 1950's. We have thus left the sentence in its original German in the main text, with an explanatory footnote in English.

missa—they are dreams that come from the gods and are consequently the real signposts of life. They are revelations. In this respect, then, the understanding of these very primitive Indians is far superior to our own. Only the ridiculous consciousness of the white man can misinterpret this by thinking that *he*—that it is *he*, *he* is the one who makes his own dreams, *he* has the ability, *he* can fabricate dreams for himself; he is the one who puts stems on all the cherries, and without *him*, they would have none.

So, just look at this mandala, which is—can you pass the book around?—this is the image of the Great Man; this is this eight-part mandala. Not one of these Indians would ever imagine that this is the ego; rather, it is the world of the Great Man. This is what the Great Man looks like. He is a symbol.

Another form that allows us to study individuation is, for example, the historical perspective—the history of the initiations, of the Mysteries. There, you will find everything, whether they are Greek or Egyptian or something else. All these symbols serve the purpose of individuation, namely, with the Great Man—to get in touch with the Great Man, and to realize his life. This is the meaning of the *imitatio Christi*; it is the meaning behind the Mysteries of an Osiris, for example. It was certainly also the meaning behind the Mysteries of Mithras, who was the god of soldiers, and who expressed the essence of the hero, which is why he was a *toreador*. You can still see this symbol alive today in the *corridas*.

On the *Puer Aeternus*

Here we have another question about the *puer aeternus*, that well-known figure in men. I have often been asked how I imagine this figure. I always reply, it is simply a metaphor to represent a certain type of behavior, a way of behaving.

Well, I should answer this in English—the *puer aeternus* is a type of behavior. It is an instinctive way of behaving, or a way of getting away with life—[Laughter] Yes, that's a type of behavior. Now the parallel figure in a woman's case is the *puella aeterna*. Of course, that is not a classical term; it's a modern parallel to the *puer aeternus*. We must realize on this occasion that psychology is recent, and in those times when the notion of the *puer aeternus* was coined, women had no psychology, you see; they were non-existent. The ancients would have been able to invent a term like *puella aeterna*, but it is not a term from antiquity. Now the *puella aeterna* is a definite figure, the eternal girl who can never die and who flourishes until 80. As a rule – not in special cases, but as a rule – the *puella aeterna* appears very late in analysis – of course, providing that the lady in question is fairly reputable. If she is not quite respectable, you know, then the *puella aeterna* can appear on the first day, but not necessarily. As a rule, one could say it takes years and years, depending on certain standards, until the *puella* appears. I have seen some most remarkable things in this respect. *Difficile est satiram non scribere.* The *puella* comes up very late and always represents a pretty difficult problem. What are the dangers the analyst must be aware of? That's a very apt question, you know, because, it's a hell of a business when you are up against it, the more respectable a lady is. Less respectable ladies are less dangerous or less of a nuisance. But the respectable lady can be a hard case because she has been repressed so long; it has been unconscious so long, and the contrast is so awful, particularly when women are old.

Our Passionate, Primitve, Chthonic, Animal Nature

This leaves us with two questions that we are coming to now, namely the question: "What is man to do with his passionate, primitive, chthonic, animal nature? In the occidental world, the chthonic passions have become identified with evil, and the spiritual passions, with good. Instead of denying them or transcending them, the psychologist may answer that we must accept the dark, instinctual forces. We must incorporate them and stop projecting them. But what does acceptance mean, and how does it make it less destructive?"[5]

This is a serious and very decisive question, one that is most frequently completely misunderstood. There is no question whether this thing could be accepted

[5] Dr. Robert Stein asks further: "Man has good reason to fear the satanic forces. It is only when they are united with the forces of light that a transformation occurs and a new creative principle is born. Perhaps this creation of the unified Godhead goes further, and it, too, must divide itself to create new passion ... new separation, union and so on. Thus, the endless cycle of birth and rebirth is perpetuated. Does this cycle continue permanently, or has man a specific role in it? Perhaps it is his uniqueness to say 'yes' and 'no'?"

or not. It cannot be accepted. That is just the trouble. It *cannot* be accepted. I mean, if you think of a very bad case of that sort, it's an impossible case; but if you analyze a case long enough, honestly and intelligently, you will come to this problem. You will come to the impossible problem. This is such a rule that I have said you cannot analyze anybody unless you come to an impossible problem, namely a problem that has no resolution [...] In such cases, one has repressed a lot of one's instinctive nature, and in analysis, of course, anybody can see how it wells up, and now we have it on the desk before us. Now what are we going to do about it? As if *we* were going to do [something] about it. Nobody can deal with it; nobody knows how to deal with it; you are absolutely lost with that problem. This must be realized first! Of course, the analysand asks, "What are you going to do about it?" I say, "Madam, I am sorry, [but] I am going to do nothing about it. I am not concerned with your damned instinctual nature. That is your business." And I would say the same to a man. I don't know! I have no prescription! What shall it be in your case? Nobody can say that. Nobody knows. Of course, for reasons of prestige, the analyst feels that he should say, "Well, you know . . ."—That's all eyewash! "Now the *puella* must be sublimated." Nobody knows how to sublimate such a thing. That's nonsense also. What *I* say to such a person is, "Go to bed now, and think of all the things you are concerned with, the unanswerable question, and see what you dream." I have no answer. Nobody has an answer. So, you [must] see how your own nature, or the unconscious, or god knows what, reacts.

Now of course, the underlying assumption of the Indians is that the Great Old Man will speak, the two-million-[year] Old Man will speak. That is a vital situation: there is an impasse; you are in a cul-de-sac, and *only then* do you hear the voice, and *it* speaks in the dream. This is the reason why we have got to understand dreams; otherwise, we never get out of this impasse. Now, you see, I'll pile [up] a mountain of symbolism and everybody swears about it. People think that by piling [up] that symbolism, I want to prove my theory. That is an awful mistake: I have amassed all of this information to give the analyst a chance to know about symbolism so that he can interpret the dreams. He must be able to interpret dreams because only dreams can answer properly—nobody else. That is just the problem: we can never answer what is to be done with this damned chthonic nature of man. The only answer is the unconscious. And then, of course, we say, "Ha, the unconscious! What should it know? What should come from there?" As if we knew. As if we knew nature. As if we knew anything about the psyche. This is damned hybris: we know nothing!

But, you see, the two-million-year Old Man, he may know something. I think that is not an exaggeration. Perhaps he has some millions, more or less, but there is a thing like nature; there is a thing like an instinctual man. If you want to know him, go to the primitives. Look at them; talk to them, then you will see it at work. Yes, I have no difficulties to talk to primitives. I can make myself understood by them very well, very easily. When I talk of the Great Man, or anything equivalent, they understand. They know that they are up against powers. We think we are on top, but that is nothing but the hybris of the city dweller. Even a peasant knows that he is up against powers. But we who live in the cities think there are no powers—well, the police, yes, or the communists or Russia, or something like that. Otherwise, we are always on top. Look at this poor chap, this man. He has foresight; it is to his great merit to have written this book. But he thinks the Great Man must be [him?].... In short, an absolute contradiction to what the Indians tell him.

There *is* the Great Man in us and that is what we call the unconscious. It is something that reacts because we *have* dreams under such conditions. Then it's up to the analyst to look at such a dream and help the patient to understand that dream. Therefore, he needs knowledge to be able to interpret what the unconscious is saying. And above all, he must have courage; for the sake of the patient, he must have the courage to believe in his own interpretation. Even if he is not quite sure, he must be able to give credit to his own interpretation. That is very difficult. When one has a critical mind, one has no end of intellectual objections to it. But, you see, it is a matter of immediate *help*! It is as if a man is bleeding to death and you stand there and deliberate [upon] which would be the best method of stopping that artery. Professor So-and-So says one has to do it this way, [while] another one says, "No, you do it that way." Well, in the meantime, that man simply pops off. That is how it is in practice, you see. I was often in the situation where I had to say, "For God's sake, I don't know. But it seems to me it is just like that." And *stand for it*! You can ask yourself in a few seconds,

"Is this really the best you could say?" When you come to the conclusion it is—by God, it is the best I can say in this case, even if I must acknowledge that somebody else might say something better. But there is no time; something must be done *now*.

Mind you, if it is an error, the unconscious will correct it. But would you believe that the unconscious can correct it, or would you think that far? Nobody thinks that the unconscious could say anything which is substantially important. Yes, one might assume, "Oh yes, it has to do with your difficulty," and so on, but, in the long run, what should the unconscious know? You must know that the process of individuation, namely that urge to become what one is, is invincibly strong. You can always count on it, and you can be sure that even if *you* are not interested in your own fate, the *unconscious* is.[...] That is difficult. It is very difficult. It is an act of courage on the part of the analyst, as well as on the part of the patient. The latter says, for instance, "Can I trust that fellow? Can I trust myself?" And the analyst thinks, "Can I trust my patient, or trust my knowledge? Perhaps my interpretation is all wrong!" He need only be sure that it is the best he can do, and mind you, it must be the best he can do. There is no cheating because that spoils the case from the beginning. You cannot cheat yourself. When you know that you have done it in a flippant and routine way, then you know that the devil is after you.

With the hybris of the intellect you get nowhere at all. So, you've got to accept what the unconscious produces, and it is up to you to understand its language. It is the language of nature. It is not your language. It is the logic of nature, the intelligence of nature, and the morality of nature that has to be translated into human forms. The form is the task, and that, you see, is the reason for the dignity of man. He makes sense in creation because, in creation, there is no reflection. Man is the one who has reflection. That is his task, and if he fulfils that task, then he can live, and he can live properly, and he is not sterilized. But when he puts himself above it, he is sterilized, stupid. It is [not] incommensurable with science. It is even the basis of science, you see. Which scientist will observe a process in nature and assume it does not exist, or that it is nothing but this or that? That's all prejudice, you see; he observes what there is. If you observe the facts that are happening in you, in reality, then you are sufficiently scientific. That is the basis of science.

The Bond Between Analysand and Analyst

Now there is another question: "Is not the *human* bond a central and vital link in analysis? I am referring to the bond between analysand and analyst."

Now I always held that the analyst is a human being, you know, belonging to the species *homo sapiens*. And so, I think a patient who thinks that his analyst is a transcendent monster and not a human thing is just a fool. But when the analyst assumes that he is transcendent and a sort of a—I don't know what—a ghost, or an abstraction, then he is the greater fool. Nobody gets out from under this fact: that he is human; and he shouldn't be ashamed of it. That is our status: we are human. So, when I talk to another human being and I am not human, that I am abstract somewhere, well, then I assume the role of God, or I don't know what. Or I think the other is a mere thought and that is also not true. So, you see, if circumstances are true and natural, the analyst is a human being and the analysand is a human being. Their Auseinandersetzung, that means a situation of dialogue, consists of two parts at least, of two human personalities. That is just so, whether one is lying on a couch covered up to the neck, and the other [is] sitting behind him, enveloped in clouds of cigar smoke. [Laughter] Both belong to the human species. [Laughter] [The] one as well as the other can be absolutely dead sure from the beginning that, in principle, each thinks the same. You see, when the patient thinks, "He is a nice man!" then the analyst probably thinks, "Isn't she a nice woman!" or something like that. If the patient thinks, "He is a disagreeable idiot!", well, then the analyst probably thinks, "Oh, damned old cat!" or something like that [Laughter], you see?

So that is the basis. A natural man, and a sound man, starts from such a natural basis. Then, having an objective situation is absolutely out of the question. That's perfectly ridiculous. It's quite impossible. Can any analyst with good sense assume that when he thinks something evil about his patient, or when the patient disgusts him, that the patient does not feel it? Of course the patient smells it, and vice versa. The thing you *are* is far stronger than your feeble words. The patient is permeated by what you are, not by what you say; he doesn't even listen to what you say. [Laughter] You see, patients listen astonishingly little and analysts all the more: but all the more... they are more permeated by the real being of the patients, and because they are analysts, they cannot admit it, because the analyst is an abstraction …in the fourth heaven, or something like that. It's all ridiculous. It's childish, simply childish. It is much better that you have a conscious conception of what you feel or what your inner thoughts are, than that you listen.

I had a patient who told me a continuous story with the greatest intensity, and she talked so much—it was of course an animus story—that for a moment I fell asleep. Then I said to her, "Did you notice?" and she said, "No, what?" I said, "Well, I just fell asleep." "Oh, did you? À *propos*, I wanted to say ..." [Laughter] *Non arrivé*! Whether I am asleep or not! Now, you see, when people are natural, they have a lot of information about other people right away. It simplifies matters considerably, but it complicates matters in as much as each has unsolved problems.

The analyst has certain unsolved problems because he is alive. He goes on living and so he must have unsolved problems, otherwise he would be dead. Life is a problem every day, and so we are never finished until we are really finished. So you see, it is quite possible that one of those problems is touched upon; it comes into play and most probably it does. This explains those cases where, very frequently—one might say it is the rule—certain analysts get certain patients which form the particular *emplastrum*[6] which they need. They get just that case which puts them up against themselves. Even if a case is not just likely to arouse a certain complex of the analyst, I am, of course, sure that, in the shortest time, each puts his foot into it. That must be so, really; this underlies human contact, and if you take it the right way, it is a most powerful means of analysis. But when you take it the wrong way, then it stops analysis, blows up everything that has been constructed. So, the analyst is [duty] bound to know about his own complexes. He shouldn't be afraid of them, and he should be able to admit that this is his prejudice when the patient gets to it.

So, you see, from a certain point on, when the patient has reached a reasonable amount of insight and a reasonable [degree of] cooperation, I do not hesitate to tell my patient, to inform my patient, that I dream of him. Because when I dream of him, he is problematic. He has touched upon something in myself where I am not the master; I am not on top

[6] Plaster, bandage.

of my own questions; I am under them, and so is he. It may be that when I tell that story to the patient, he says, "Ah yes, that's it. I have dreamt so and so!", and he brings me a dream that elucidates my own problem. That means we have now reached a place where I might be profiting from that analysis, [where I am] helped with my own problems, and I help the other. I call it the *paternoster* work of—[do] you know what that is, *paternoster* work? In the old mines where they had no lifts yet, they had long ladders that always moved in this way. So, you stepped on the one and then when the other ladder came up, you stepped upon that and then you stepped upon another one, and that's how you got up very quickly, on those two ladders that simply moved like this. That is *paternoster* work.

So, you see, each step forward that the patient makes can be a step forward for the analyst, too. That is human intercourse; you cannot be with somebody without being completely permeated by that other person. But [if] you don't notice it, [if] you don't know this, you will say things that belong to another psychology, not your own, and a certain atmosphere will take hold of you and will increase or decrease your own prejudices. And so, when you analyze a patient for any length of time, something of that kind will occur. Then you must be wise. You must know where you are, and you have to share certain, perhaps very private, opinions, judgments, and moods etc. When a patient says, "Oh doctor, it's too bad that you are in a bad mood today," then you say, "Oh, not at all, not at all," because you were not able to acknowledge your own condition. That's a point against you. I think it is a point against a patient who's fairly advanced [when I say], "Now how is it with you today? You look funny!" "Oh, I'm not funny at all! I'm perfectly normal." Now that doesn't hold water, you know. Then out comes the story that *should* be *said*—particularly important with feeling types. With feeling types, you have to enquire every day, "Now what. . .?"—about the weather, practically: "How do you feel? How do I appear to you? What kind of feelings have you about me? What things are you chewing over?", you know, to keep abreast. Because, you see, for an intellectual, the feeling type is a thorny type because, time and again, they touch on his own deficiencies. The analyst is unaware of his feelings; he doesn't realize what his feelings are—while the other is all the time *au courant*—and is looking at his cards, and that is not profitable. Not at all. That is all the ordinary forms of inferiorities, or inferior functions, you know.

[Question:] "Does not the stress on 'transference analysis' obviate the possibility of the analyst functioning in the capacities of a shaman, or medicine man, or psychopompos?"

[C.G. Jung:] I hope he is hindered as much as possible! You see, that is exactly why one has transference analysis, meaning the business of transference understood as a sort of projection that is hindering the clear understanding of the situation.

Now one of the greatest hindrances to [having] a clear understanding is the projection of the shaman, of the psychopompos, of the medicine man, the spiritual doctor, of the great spirit, I don't know what, the saviour. As soon as you are elevated to such a rank, you are made powerless! [...] Then the analyst is a fool; he is completely blindfolded, and he is lost in a sea of mist. So, whenever signs appear of such an archetype—an archetypical projection—that is a warning. You say then at once, "For heaven's sake, do you think I am a shaman or something like that?" That must be discouraged as soon as possible because it is an archetype, and then the archetype rules over the situation. The analyst is in the role of the archetype: he is then back to being the shaman, and then he is just as unable to work miracles as the shaman is as a rule. He is absolutely hindered, and every proposal of life is obviated completely. But when that thing is analyzed—for example the father complex, you see, which is at the bottom of it and raises the analyst to the role of a demigod [and] of course, that must be analyzed; of course, that must be reduced to human size—there is still the human being. That is not the whole of transference. That would be simple, you know; you could give it to the patient in the form of a printed form and you sign that form: "I declare I am no shaman. I am not God. I am not Christ. I am no savior. I am not this nor that," and I [could] hand it to the patient, and he countersigns it. Then you're OK. But you see, the transference is a living thing. It may appear in the form of a father transference, or a Christ transference, or anything of the sort. And that is a mistake; it is a deviation which is not proceeding [from], or produced by, the bad will of the patient, but by his perplexity. He doesn't know what that other fellow is: is he perhaps Jesus Christ, or is he the Buddha, or is he a shaman or something like that? It is an unhappy word he uses for lack of the right word. He doesn't know what [he is dealing with].

On the other hand, if he were a Naskapi, he would say, "Oh I know, that's his Great Man, or her Great Man." Then he would have the formula, "Now I see: he is the Great Man, and have I not such a Great Man also? Is this perhaps the business between two Great Men, not between Mr. So-and-so and Mr. So-and-so or Mrs. So-and-so?" The Naskapi would have a great advantage. It is a mountain of work until people can see this, and how many of the analysts of today understand it? Very few, I tell you. But that is the point in analysis, you see? At first it seems [the analyst] is the good papa, or the bad papa, and then he is this and that and so on—a whole series of things, all [of which] are attempts at qualifying the riddle, to see the enigma; and it is vital to the patient that he finds out about it. Because if he does not find it out with the analyst, he cannot find it out with himself. There is nobody else who would listen to him, so it must be the analyst. The analyst must be able to answer these questions so that the patient can see what he or she is. Unless you can compare yourself with something, you cannot say "I am this and not that." So, he must be able to say, "I am this," but he can only say this when he knows what the facts are. That is the purpose of this form of transference.

Then let us assume we have come to the end of these perplexities, and there is still the question of transference, still the same thing, and we have no name for it; then it must be quite personal. That is awkward because both know it isn't [personal]. If they are honest, it isn't. It's something else. Everyone who is convinced that there is an unconscious and there is such a thing as archetypes, well, he is to be congratulated because he knows what it is. He knows, "Ah, here is an archetype at play, and it is the Great Man," or whatever he calls the thing behind the scenes. And then he discovers that, at bottom, transference is by no means a personal fantasy that has to be reduced. You lose an enormous value when you reduce it to a personality, to an individual personality. It may be that you used it in connection with the collective unconscious, with the real source of life. So, if you are wise, you must teach your patient about the double possibility man has, namely, to be entirely personal, which is in no way different from an animal; or that he assumes that there is something more than human personality, namely the Great Man, or something of the sort, which is the prerogative of man. Then he can see the situation in another light. You only arrive at this insight by dream analysis and by understanding symbolism. That is what makes it so difficult.

On Medical Training

There is only one further question and that is a very practical question concerning "the medical training of analysts, or the measures that could be taken at universities to give medical students a concept of the psychological aspect of disease."[7]

That is the big question. There is no real method in this respect yet. There are only individual experiments at various universities.

[. . .]

[7] Dr. Helene Hoffmann; "In your opinion, what observations suggest that medical education in Europe has already received stimulation and benefits from your creative life's work? What measures within medical studies could you suggest to facilitate a student's access to his or her own inner world, something so essential for the physician?"

I have had the most incredible experiences in this regard, and I am utterly disappointed in this matter. One could achieve it by designating a faculty to hold lectures about it, to establish a chair for it. But then, of course, someone will be chosen who knows as little as it is possible to know. I have witnessed this: it was once discussed here whether one could create a chair for psychotherapy, and suggestions were made. I heard about it indirectly. And the one who was nominated [...], the candidate for this vice-chancellorship, was the youngest and the stupidest student in my seminar. He didn't even finish his analysis, but dropped out before it was over because he couldn't understand that the unconscious is not conscious. [Laughter] Since then, nothing has happened. In any event, I wouldn't have been accepted here, certainly not at a Swiss university—that would have been impossible. That's one of the main reasons why things aren't moving forward, of course, because a selection committee naturally selects according to the bottom line, and nothing … well, I can't think of anything that could be done in a general way in this area. So much depends on the local circumstances that you can't say anything general. And I cannot claim that European medical training has been influenced in any way by my life's work.

You know, Freud said something quite similar at the end of his life, namely that his psychoanalysis was much less suited to physicians than to other people. The psychological standpoint is not very important to today's physicians, although I know many physicians who are very interested in it; in the upper echelons, however, they have no say in this matter. And physicians are not particularly bad people in this respect but are simply like all other people who have terrible resistances. For example, they think I'm bald and yet I'm supposed to have beautiful white curls down to my shoulders and big blue eyes and a beautiful white beard—this repugnant guy. This is what the psychologist looks like. Indeed, things will go on this way for quite some time, and if these basic facts of the human mind are not even understood in psychological circles, so that one does not even know what the anima is, and such things, we cannot possibly speak of wanting to educate doctors in general.

On the Practice of Analysis

[C.G. Jung:] The first question I would like to deal with is Dr. Marie-Louise von Franz's question, which will not take us long. It's a question that has plagued many an analyst, namely: "When should I intervene, or should I intervene at all, in an ongoing analysis?"

If you want to do psychology, I recommend taking note of something the philosopher Multatuli said—well, his pseudonym is Multatuli. He once said: "Nothing is completely true, and even that is not completely true." You need to get that through your head! There are rules, and there are no rules. Every sentence in psychology can be reversed and it will still be right, or only then is it right; it all depends on the circumstances, which are sometimes completely imponderable. And the final call on difficult issues does not reside in the head or in the heart, but somewhere in that psychological no-man's land where you don't know where it's coming from. In those instances, it may be an act of fate or an act of grace, or it may be a helpful kind of malice that comes to the rescue.

As a rule, it is certainly true that we should not intervene, because when we intervene with our naive mindset, there are a whole lot of assumptions and projections involved, of which we are not aware. So be cautious about intervening. And then suddenly you find yourself in a situation where, bearing this principle in mind, you think, "Yes, I shouldn't intervene," when in fact you would have intervened, and it would have been the right thing to do. A patient may say to you a long time after the fact, "But for heaven's sake, why didn't you tell me at the time? You knew, so how could you sit there without batting an eye and leave me to stew in my nonsense?" You see, then, don't you, what a mistake you perhaps made? You observed a law, or a rule, and you didn't look at the case in hand—and you didn't look at yourself while doing so. You must at least ask yourself, if I am to take this patient seriously and I really want to help them, how do I react to this? You must identify with them as much as possible and ask yourself, "How would *I* act in this situation?" Only if you think like that and are so minded, will the patient realize that you really care about their situation, as if it were really the analyst's own business. Then, if they feel that commitment, they are more likely to listen to your advice, and you are more likely to be able to intervene.

I once had a case of an elderly doctor; she was about 56, and she came to me in a state of complete *Amentia*, that is, in a confused state of mind. At the time, I said, "Good heavens, what has happened to you? What is the matter with you?" It turned out she had been in a Freudian analysis where she had had to lie on the couch, and the analyst had sat down behind her, hoping nothing could get to him, and simply didn't respond. She then fantasized out loud to no one in particular, and she tried to shock him, to upset him, to get some kind of reaction from this blockhead, for heaven's sake, and nothing came – with the result that she became more and more crazy. In the end, she had to stop her analysis, for she felt she was becoming utterly confused. That's just … I mean, for God's sake, that is just an inhumane way of behaving! And then she said, "Look, you're having an affect!" And I said, "Yes, of course I'm having an affect. What do you imagine? Do you believe I am a blockhead? I am not a…not a theoretically stunted, pathetic creature, devoid of almost all human reactions." If I am having an affect, then I am having an affect. And I've shown that to people on occasion—indeed, I have—that I'm having an affect. [Laughter.] I don't want to tell you everything I did in this case. But in this way, you cut years off an analysis.

This one hour sufficed to reestablish this woman's sound mind. Of course, she is going to lose her orientation if the analyst does not react, or if he does not say what he thinks about the situation. When someone comes with a crazy plan, where you see that everything [...] [has] come together in a conspiracy to destroy him, and you say nothing, that's inhumane, isn't it? On the other hand, you can help the patient with their active imaginations: You should put yourself inside these fantasies and not stand by like a chump, but take part in them. But when the analyst does not participate, he is doing precisely what he told his patient not to do. And always …this is completely stupid, this kind of thing; it just shows that the analyst can't be natural, and if he can't be natural, he should call it quits from the start.

Mind you, it can happen that you have the feeling "Yes, now one should..." and you do not know what one should do. But if you ask yourself what you should do with this case right now, you can state quite openly that you are stupid, and say, "I don't know, I don't know what to do about it." At the very least, you can show that you're with them on the journey; that if you knew what to do, you would do it. It has happened to me over and over again that I have not understood a dream. Then instead of making a grandiose face, I say: [Laughter]. "I'm sorry, I don't understand this dream, I don't know what it means."

So that's the situation with intervention. You may find yourself in a situation where, for humane reasons, you have to say something, perhaps even something very cutting. Not because of theoretical considerations, mind you, which don't count, but because of the human situation. This is decided solely by your instinct; you must make sure that you are at one with your instinct. That is what decides, not your good intentions and not theoretical considerations or so-called insights into the structure of neurosis: none of that will help you. The wholeness of one's personality, which is ineffable, will help you at this moment—if you have not thoroughly offended it beforehand. Do you have any questions about this?

- Yes, please?

[Question:] I would like to ask you, Professor Jung, you said that at the moment you intervene, you risk, at least, that you are also projecting a lot of things or are somehow unconscious about your own affect, and so on. So, what then is the attitude of the analyst after intervening in an affect? In this kind of intervention, a part of your unconscious is in the shadow, for example, which, in this instance, means it has been brought into direct contact with the patient. Then, of course, an analyst must be ready to discuss this.

[C.G. Jung:] Yes, naturally, of course.

[Question:] That he has had an affect.

[C.G. Jung:] Yes, of course, and why he's having an affect, so that the patient can get his bearings; otherwise, it is not a discussion; otherwise, the analyst is sitting in a cloud, thinking that he is invisible, and the patient is left clueless. Of course, he must answer the patient's questions; the latter should be treated as a human being and not as some poor sick person one is taking care of. This is a completely disgusting attitude; even if they are ill, they should be seen as a human being.

On the Nature of Guilt

[C.G. Jung:] Dr. Hess's question is a longer discourse on the nature of guilt, which I shall not read aloud. There are people who experience guilt, and others who don't experience guilt. And [therefore] one question is: "Is guilt possible where there is not yet an ego?" […]

So, on the principle of the concept of guilt: If you consult, for example, criminal law about what is understood by guilt—you can also consult the Catholic practice of confession—you will hear that there is no guilt where there is no ego, i.e., where no one was present, where people are simply unconscious of having done something evil, or the like. This is not the case in nature; there all guilt on earth is avenged. One is treated mercilessly by nature, as if one really were guilty. So, for example, if you have never heard of bacteria or that there is contaminated water, and you just drink any water and you get typhoid fever, that is how nature treats you, as I just indicated.

Nature doesn't ask if you know; it just does it, and you are the fool. Whereas human law, or even the moral law of the Church, asks whether one is conscious of guilt. So, for example, I remember a rather blatant case where a grand lady went to a Jesuit priest to have her confession heard. He was a very shrewd man and she intended to confess certain delicate situations of her life to him. And after she had finished with her normal confession and then wanted to confess the above, which wasn't quite according to the rule, he stopped her and asked, "Excuse me, but is what you're about to say something that you feel guilty about?" And then, seeing the light, she said, "Well, not really." "Then there is no need for you to confess it, madam." [Laughter.]

So that's roughly how you can put this point of view to use. But nature shows no mercy: it punishes those who are unconscious just as much, and perhaps even more, than those who know. So, guilt is—if we speak of it in human terms—a consciousness; it's a conscious guilt, which doesn't exist, of course, where there is no ego. But even where there is no ego, there can still be guilt. The Indians express this by saying that one is subject to karma. Now, this karma can be of a personal nature; one knows, "This is my karma."

Or it is an impersonal karma, which one…which the mother….which, when one was swimming in one's mother's womb, one picked up somewhere, because it was floating around. The Indian doctrine of karma is not clear in this respect.

These considerations are also valid in the case where the ego, an ego, is present, but it happens to be unconscious of any guilt. This is then the same as before: there is no ego for this guilt. There is no one to take on this guilt. Now, no matter how this guilt is incurred, whether by this or by that, by being lazy or by being pedantic or clever, it is of no consequence in this regard. It is just a question of whether such a burden is consciously or unconsciously present. The most dangerous forms are, of course, the unconscious ones, because nature is cruel in this respect. I mean, nature does not judge like a judge; it simply implements consequences, and we can only blame ourselves for that and realize that we are the stupid ones—the foolish, stupid, and unconscious worms that humans are, you see? And hence we have the Hermetic tenet: the demiurge has created a world, which is highly imperfect, and people, who can only crawl on all fours. Then, however, the higher God of the spiritual worlds took pity on these worms and sent them a *krater*[8] which is filled with *nous*[9] for the unconscious ones to bathe in. Thus, the better among them noticed that there was something going on. This question was, in fact, discussed even at that time. It's true, isn't it, that the well-known Greek quotation "*pothen to kakon*"[10] comes from a Gnostic. They were dealing with these problems.

Today, we can understand why the Gnostics were so extremely troublesome for the Church: they were discussing the very problems that the Church had failed to answer. For the Church knows nothing of any guilt we are burdened with about which we know nothing. Of course, one can draw far too broad a conclusion out of sheer lack of instinct and say, "Yes, I'm to blame for everything." For example, you are not to blame that there are typhoid bacilli in this water. But if you have once had the opportunity to read in the newspaper that there is infected drinking water, and you do not remember it, then you are in error—the fault lies with you; you have not drawn any conclusions. But if you have never heard that

[8] A vessel to mix wine in.
[9] Mind, reason, spirit.
[10] Where does evil come from?

there are bacteria that could be infecting the drinking water, and you drink the water, then, of course, in human terms, you are completely innocent. But in the eyes of nature, you are to blame. And that is how our whole life is: in the eyes of nature, we are to blame, for we have not yet reached that level of awareness we need to reach, for which humankind has actually been created. We have not yet achieved it. We are still unconscious in too many respects, and this is quite glaring. You see the difference every day when you compare what you know about [our psychological] background and what lay people know: you have a wider consciousness. So, what you achieve through psychology is a more expanded consciousness. And you should not abuse it and draw delusory conclusions that you are to blame for everything, or that you bear the sins of the world. We are not gods; we are simply still too unconscious. We are only at the beginning of any real consciousness. Thus, there should not be any instance of people who could know, simply not giving the thing in question any consideration, or choosing not to think about such things out of stupid naivety or laziness.

I remember the case of a professor of theology: When I wrote my book *Wandlungen und Symbole der Libido*

(Transformations and Symbols of the Libido), he wrote a very unpleasant critique about it in which he reproached me that—*en flagrant contradiction avec la parole du Maitre*[11]—I had said that one may not remain a child, but rather one must become an adult. [Laughter] This miserable fool didn't even notice the passage in St. Paul where he talks about giving up our childish ways—that one must first be an adult to become a child once again. Christ did not say, "Ye shall remain children," but rather "become like children." This professor had not understood this. He hadn't given it a thought, but then accuses me of claiming, in flagrant opposition to Christ's words, that one must do away with one's childish ways, that one cannot remain infantile, when, in fact, you know, the ideal is for one to uphold one's childlike faith.

He was a Protestant. I could tell you an identical story about a learned Jesuit priest who indignantly sought me out. He had read my *Job*, and he had only one question about it, and that was: "What makes you state that Christ and Mary were not human beings?" [Then I said]: "Well, my dear professor, that is terribly simple; I don't see why you would

[11] In flagrant contradiction with the Master's word.

ask me that. After all, according to your own dogma, you were born in original sin. You bear the *macula peccati,*[12] as do I; all humans are corruptible and corrupted, which is why we die—we are mortal. [This is] just basic knowledge, the consequences of the *macula peccati*. But what about Christ and Mary? They are in the condition of innocence, the original innocence, namely in the *status gratiae*[13] before original sin, which means they are uncorrupted; which is why, isn't it, that Christ also went to heaven with his body—of course, with a glorified body. And the same is true of Mother Mary. They are not people; they are gods." This man, who was certainly an intelligent man, had never thought of that. He was completely perplexed by what is a very simple conclusion; there's nothing to it at all. He had no answer.

Look, I mean, all these types of unconsciousness, they of course take wretched revenge. For him, a highly intellectual man compared to a physician, that was a damnable defeat. I never saw him again. [Laughter]

[12] The stain of sin.

[13] State of grace.

So, guilt doesn't go only as far as we acknowledge it; it goes much further. This natural guilt, I don't know how far it goes; I don't know how great the commitments are that we made when we were born, and for which we have, or bear, no guilt.

Body and Mental Development

Let's go on to the next question. It is a question from Mr. Hillman. Well, this question has to do with the importance of the body as the basis of the psychic process. The question, if I understand it properly, seems to be whether the body is the apt vessel or is a good vessel for mental development or the mental process. The question Mr. Hillman puts at the end is, "What can we do towards strengthening and refining the vessel? How can we bring ourselves and our patients closer to an incarnation of the process and the resurrection of the flesh?"

I would say, "According to my bias and to the resurrection of the spirit." [Jung laughs.] Now I should be grateful to Mr. Hillmann if he would kindly explain a little bit, or comment on his question so that I see more clearly what it is about.

[J. Hillmann:] I think I said in the first paragraph that after a certain stage in the process is arrived at, where the dynamic content or the spirit shows itself, a lot depends on the body as the vessel for holding this—and often the ...

[C.G. Jung:] Ah yes, there you say it—excuse me when I interrupt you. "As the analysis proceeds, so that a certain access to the spirit has been made possible and dynamic contents have begun to move, the whole trick of the work seems to depend upon the vessel. Without it being ripe, the process never becomes real, or it just goes up in the air, or it can turn and destroy."

All this is perfectly true, but think, for instance, of people who are in a serious physical predicament, that means gravely ill, perhaps even dying, where the body is really seriously in question. Yet it is the only moment in the life of that fellow where some spiritual or psychical process is possible at all. And his body is not at all in a favorable condition—quite the contrary. You see, certain people need, for instance, a physiological illness in order to be able to understand something of psychology. Only when they are ill or in pain are they apt to understand some psychological connection or [something] of psychological significance. As long as they are normal, they are as dull as stones; nothing registers. Sure enough, one always says "*In corpore sano mens sana,*" that the mind is sound in a sound body. That is a general truth, but don't forget the psychological device: nothing is true, and even that is not quite true.

So, you see, one can have a perfectly splendid mental or spiritual state, despite the body. Indeed, the one who is wounded can heal the wound, and the one who is handicapped by his body can develop arts and crafts or ideas which other people cannot do.

So, the general banal truth which you can read in *Reader's Digest* [laughter] for instance, is that you must have a healthy body and then everything is all right. While that is generally true, this sentence is so hellishly banal that it must also be true when you turn it round: you don't need a healthy body in order to be mentally sane or advanced even. On the contrary! But there is also an unsound attitude of neglecting the body, of thinking derogatory things about the body. One shouldn't do such foolish things; one should give everything its due value. When you see an ass, a donkey, and you think, "Aha, this is an ass, a terribly stupid animal," you are making a mistake: the ass is not a stupid animal. It is the same as if you were thinking of Mr. So-and-So with whom you have dealings, and you think, "Of course, he is an ass." He is not necessarily an ass. Or you think, "He is a liar," when he is not necessarily a liar. If you think he is a liar and treat him as such, then you are the stupid ass who is making a bad mistake because you cannot deal with him. So, when you think the wrong thing about anything, you are the idiot who is turning something perfectly all right into nonsense by your projection. The same thing can be done with the body: there are plenty of people [...] who neglect their body, and that is naturally based upon a certain resistance to the body, or even a philosophic or religious bias concerning the body, and then I interfere. I say, "Now, look here! You cannot neglect yourself like that. It shows that you have foolish resistances." And later on, they will say they were ever so grateful to me that I mentioned this thing because they had been keeping it under their hat. Stefan Georg was just such a fellow. When he came to the hospital in Bâle, he was lousy with dirt, incredible. Or Thomas Becket, the Archbishop of Canterbury who was murdered, had eczema all over his body; he was terribly dirty and neglected. That is, of course, a useless prejudice, and it is against instinct; here, too, one must simply have the right instinct. Of course, that's easily said but most difficult to do. But when you feel with the patient, you get a certain notion: "Ah, that fellow is on the wrong track somewhere." You can apply the same technique to yourself and realize that you eat too much or too little, or that you eat the wrong thing and are constipated, and such things. It is pathological when people simply neglect themselves in this respect; it is part of a neurosis, or very often the outcome of a historical bias. Of course, we shouldn't be so corporeal; one should be spiritual and then one doesn't eat, or develops an ulcer, and then it is much better! Have you got anything to ask about that?

Well, you see, I must say I see no problem here: why shouldn't we admire the beauty of the body? The body can be very beautiful. [...]

About Rituals

Now here is a question from Mr. Stein: "How can we, who, through your works and your spirit, have found a way back to ourselves and the source, find a vessel to receive it in the outer collective? Must we resort to the use of traditional rituals, and hope that the living God will once more make them alive, or are we destined to wait until there are new bottles—no, skins really—to contain the new wine? If so, what happens in the meantime? The individual cannot hold too much of the spirit without losing consciousness. And finally, I ask: Can the individual really maintain a relationship to the self if there are no traditional rituals which enable him to return from his night sea journey?"

Well, I must say, somebody who lives in the present time and has a certain psychological understanding, and who finds nothing more threatening than rituals because they take him right back into the past, hasn't understood. For example, how can we assume that a living god needs a church? If he cannot manifest without a church, that thing is very suspect. Such a god would mean damn little to me.

You see, it is not a question of finding a vessel: *we are* the vessel; *we are* the instrument, and if we don't function as such, then we have no spirit. Because the experience of a man with spirit is that he is made to function. That makes him tick. He doesn't question whether there is a collective form in which he could express himself. That means he needs consciousness. He *cannot* function, so he needs a ritual. You see, *if* the spirit wants a ritual, *you* will do it; if it does not want a ritual, no ritual on earth can replace the spirit.

There is no substitute for the spirit, and somebody who seeks a ritual, well, that's simply a declaration that he cannot be, and he cannot function without being contained. That is like a child who says, "I can't walk, unless my mother holds me." Well, that is not a proper function: that is a paralysis.

The traditional ritual helps us to remain in contact with the self as *we* understand it. It helps you to remain in contact with an idea, a symbolic idea, that we declare to have been an idea of the self. For instance, *we* say that Christ in a certain way is the idea of the *homo maximus*, of the *anthropos*, of the *filius hominis*. That is a symbol of the self. But in as much as we have the idea that Christ really means the self, that very same ritual becomes the worst temptation to lose your relation to the self. For instance, if you are a bit sensitive and you go to a beautiful mass, you go into that beautiful ritual, and you forget yourself; you're dissolved into that beautiful form, but it doesn't help you to keep any relation to yourself. To keep to the self is an intimate, individual experience and an intimate, individual activity, an effort where anything, even if it is something very spiritual, will be a mere hindrance that hinders you from understanding or becoming aware of your relatedness to the self. The self is in that respect a very small, tiny, and very tender thing that cannot be disturbed by outside influences. So, you see, a man who is all alone by himself and has no church, no holy water, and no communion would be quite lost. Such a person has no relation to the self. One's relation to the self is in the first place a lonely experience, and only in as much as you find understanding or people with similar experiences are you not isolated. But it doesn't help you to go to church or to follow certain rituals to get that feeling because you won't get it.

I once knew an old Catholic peasant [who] said to me, "Doctor, you know so many things. I would like you to once explain to me why we Catholics do not stick together?" I said, "But don't you stick together?" He said, "Oh no, we don't stick together. The Protestants are far more interested in each other."

He gave me examples in a very naive way and then I saw what he meant. He meant something quite intelligent: the Protestant has no ritual, practically; he has no community in a form. If there is community, it is all human and often quite rational. But in Catholicism, it is quite different: you have a church; you are a member of the Church; you are in the Church; and that is your relationship to other people. You don't need to take care of it. If you go through Protestant villages, the dung heaps are neatly folded, and they are quite a sight. In Catholic villages, the dung heap is very often not nice; it's in a rather bad and unaesthetic state. You can see these things because the Catholics care less about what other people think. The Protestant is far more concerned with his neighbors.

A parson here in Zurich told me an interesting story. A shoemaker, who was a Czechoslovakian Catholic, brought his seven children to him to be confirmed. He got interested and went to that man and asked him, "I know you and your wife are Catholic, so why do you send your children to me?" He said, "Well, I know it's very peculiar, but I think it's better for them; they'll learn more about social connections and friendships than if they are Catholic. Because in a way we [Catholics] get off too easily with confession; it takes the sting out of things, and then why go any further? Why make an effort?"

You see, that is a very serious thing. For instance, I had a colleague who was a professor, a medical man like me, and he once asked me, "Now tell me, what would you call a neurosis?" Of course, I was careful not to say, "Why do you have to know?" I explained to him carefully what a neurosis is. He thought a while and then he said, "Well, if that is so then about two thirds of my clientele are neurotic." Then I said, "Very likely so." Then he said, "I don't see why you are so interested in psychology and why you take such immense trouble to understand these things. You see, when I am in trouble or if I have a problem, I ask my father confessor. If he doesn't know a solution, he asks the bishop, and if the bishop has no solution, he writes to Rome where, for two thousand years, the most intelligent people have been sitting together, and they have worked out these problems long ago. [Laughter] Why are you interested in the human mind? It has all been done, and this is now a form, you know, this *Roma locuta; causa finite*."[14] That is ritual; that is ritual life for you.

Now such a man, you see, hasn't even an interest; he sees nothing; he is completely blind. If fate had thrown me together with him—and he is a nice fellow and I should have been a friend of his—I would have been a white elephant to him forever. He would have understood nothing at all, and I would have handled him like a sack of potatoes. Because such a man means nothing to me whatsoever. It is a serious handicap to live in a ceremonial or ritualistic way. The vessel grasps for you; you don't grasp.

[14] Rome has spoken; the cause is ended.

God-Image and the Self

[C.G. Jung:] The next [question] is [from] Mr. Dreifuss about the God-image. Here I shall answer in German. His question arose from a passage in my work on Job, where I say that humankind has an infinitely small but more concentrated light than the God of creation. Accordingly, the human being or human consciousness has a more concentrated light than God, or the image of God. Since we have only an image; we talk about the images, about the psychology of the image. But what God himself is, we don't know; that is something ineffable, an *arrheton.*[15] Mr. Dreifuss asks the question: "To what extent is the ego greater than the self? Is not the image of God always more extensive than human consciousness?"

Well, this question does not necessarily follow from that. You can have a more concentrated image of something within the circumference of the self, can't you? The ego is within the circumference of the self. It's a smaller self perhaps, and the smaller it

[15] Unspoken.

is, the more acute is its light, the more concentrated its light. The image in question—the self—is so difficult to realize because it is so vague; it can best be compared to a twilight, even though at times it may seem to us the most concentrated of lights. In its illumination . . .think of the illuminations of the saints, where a tremendous light breaks in on them; it is nevertheless [...]. Wherever we encounter this idea of the self, it is difficult for us to grasp; it is also something—and you know this from your own experience—that is difficult to realize, for its nature is that of a totality, to which our nature, of course, does not correspond.

How can we be whole? We are born specialized, as it were. One person is born with a good mind, while another is born with a good heart; a third spends their entire life simply taking things in and has neither a heart nor a mind. All these various preconditions imply just as many limitations. The desire, then, on the part of the self to realize itself is up against a great obstacle. Theoretically speaking, it is actually impossible for the self to realize itself; it can only happen gradually. We have no idea to what degree it has been realized, or whether it has been realized at all, or how much of it has been realized: we have no measure. We know from what is realized in us that it always transcends our boundaries.

Whatever wants to become realized in you creates, for example, an inflation, an overestimation of yourself, or an underestimation of yourself. It disturbs. This is why we are so afraid of individuation. People are *afraid* of themselves, and that is why they don't want to know anything about the unconscious. They are afraid that something will come that they can't control, or not very well, or that they will have the greatest difficulty even forming an idea of what it is. It presents us with outrageous tasks, and then, of course, you ask yourself, "What *is* this thing?" And, in the same way when you think of another person and ask yourself "What is he like, what qualities does he have, I mean, what are his values?" So, too, you ask yourself about the self. Then you discover that however far it extends upwards, the self also extends downwards, which now makes it really scary, for not only what is good gains entry through the self, but also what is evil. If a *person* were like the self, people would say, "Oh yes, they contradict themselves constantly; they are utterly confused!" Right now, at this moment, the self seems as high as possible, and then, in the next moment, it seems as low as possible, and you simply can't fathom it. What tremendous difficulty people have to grasp that the God-image is ambivalent. Now in the Bible it is written that it is [like that], and you can read it there. But it *may* not be thus, it may not be thus.

Asian cultures, however, have been able to grasp this; they have grasped that the gods have a benevolent and a malevolent appearance. Thus, the lovely Kuan-Yin, for example, when she gives the evil spirits in hell their daily food, she appears in the form of an evil spirit, for she is so good, she doesn't want to scare the evil spirits. Think of Mother Mary feeding the evil spirits in hell and putting on a fur pelt with a tail on it. [Laughter] Hardly!

The self is, in fact, like some Japanese woodblock prints I saw: hell is at the bottom with Kuan-Yin going about as a terrible ghost, looking devilish. She moves around as a devil and feeds the evil spirits, as it were. And from her head a thin thread reaches far up into the sky, and there is tiny little Kuan-Yin seated on her throne in the silver moonlight, as a faint memory, when in fact, right now, she is the evil demon.

The East is able to think concurrently about this. I think I have told you the story—a trick question from India. Somebody asked me, "What do you think? Who takes longer to see God: the one who loves Him or the one who hates Him?" You see, there are the two opposites being thought simultaneously in a way that we in the West cannot do. Even the theologians, who ought to know the most about what God can do [...]. They are so prejudiced, it is impossible for them to think like that. But what we know from the psychology of the unconscious is that the self is utterly contradictory. And it is so in a manner that simply confounds us. You realize, "Yes. This is beyond me." And if the circumstances require it, you may have a dream which is very important and which tells you a highly paradoxical truth, one that, with the best will in the world, you cannot grasp. Is this some form of devilry, or supreme spirituality, or what? It is just antonymous, and therefore the image of God is transcendent, because it eludes our grasp.

This image of the self that we have within us is always symbolized—not by us, but historically speaking—as a god. It is, after all, an image of God, and an image of the soul. So, for example, *deus est circulus cuius centrum est ubique circumferentia vero nusquam*: God is a circle whose center is everywhere, and whose circumference is nowhere. This image also holds true of the soul. The soul was imagined as a round sphere or as a circle—and these are the symbols that we also encounter within our psychology. Now this indicates that the self, the image of the self, the concept of the self that we have formed, is an analogy, an *analogia dei*. It's an image of God; we can't get around that. Now, all qualities which we can determine empirically ourselves are also statements of a transcendental nature; they are statements made about the highest being i.e., of the uttermost being. And about this, we can only speak in contradictory terms.

BIBLIOGRAPHY

Jung, C.G. (1964). *Collected Works, Volume 10*. Edited and translated by G. Adler, R. F.C. Hull. Princeton, NJ: Princeton University Press.

Nietzsche, F. (1886). *Beyond Good and Evil*. Leipzig: C.G. Naumann.

Speck, F.G. (1935). *Naskapi: The Savage Hunters of the Labrador Peninsula*. Norman, Oklahoma: University of Oklahoma Press.

Made in United States
North Haven, CT
04 November 2026

21766926R00067